Child Care & Training Booklets

The Rewards of Right Eating

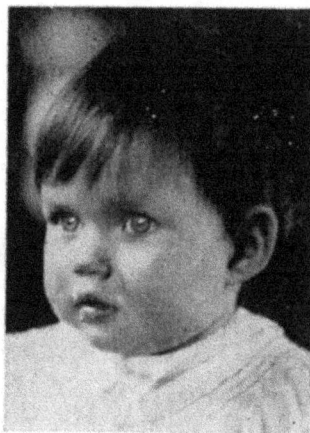

IOWA STATE COLLEGE
EXTENSION SERVICE

The Rewards of Right Eating

BY MRS. ALMA H. JONES

"Of the three necessities of life which the home must provide, food, clothing and shelter, food is the most important. Without it, life is impossible. With scanty provision, growth is stunted and power declines. With abundance, one may stuff the furnace until the fires of life are dulled by sheer surplus of good fuel. By indiscreet choice, precious days of life may be lost by headaches or other acute, tho minor, ills, and by continued bad feeding the way is paved for serious impairment of health. For food, people spend the largest part of their incomes. What a pity if they buy sickness instead of health!"*

*Mary Schwartz Rose, Ph.D.; Feeding the Family. Introduction.

I. Is Health or Sickness Purchased with the Food Which We Buy?

Do the market baskets of America bring health or illness into the homes which they supply with food? If we base our answer on data regarding health conditions existing with American school children, we conclude that too often the market basket contributes to defects and illness instead of abounding health and vigor. It is estimated that 75 percent of American school children have physical defects of various kinds, the most common defects being:

> 50-90 percent have decayed teeth
> 30-40 percent have adenoids and diseased tonsils
> 25-40 percent have defects of posture and foot arches
> 15-25 percent are malnourished

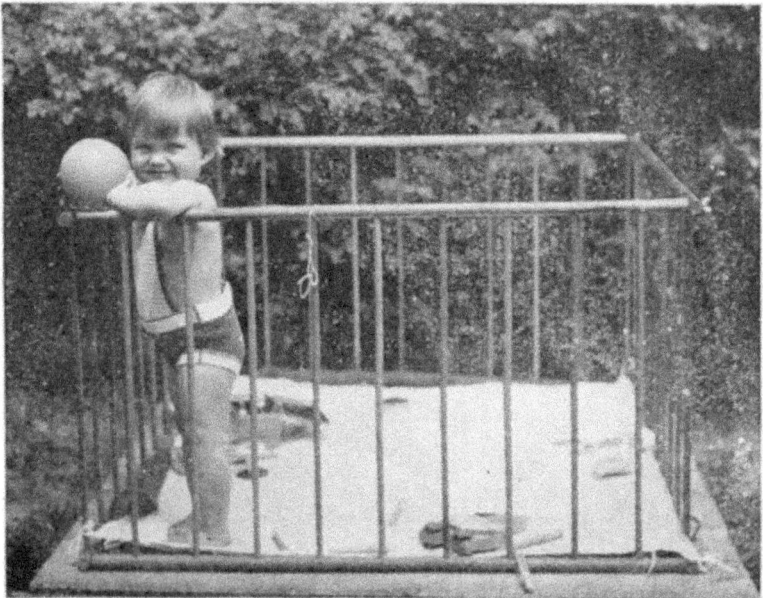

Fig. 1. Evidence of optimal health in babyhood. (Note sun-suit.)

The common physical defects of children are usually attributed to the following causes:

Insufficient and improper diet and faulty food habits.

Over-fatigue and insufficient sleep.

Unpleasant and irritating home conditions.

Faulty health habits.

Since diet is such a large factor in the prevention of the various physical defects of childhood, it is evident that sickness and not health is often purchased with the food which we buy.

The purpose of this booklet is to show what is meant by a well child and to show that proper f o o d i s conducive to optimum health and fitness in children.

II.   What is a Well Child?

Someone has said that the well child is a "growing, going and glowing child."

By a well child we do not mean one that is temporarily free from illness or disease, or one which is free from glaring physical defects, as may be the case with "average" children.   The well child is one that shows growth, development and functioning of the body as "optimal" or at its best.

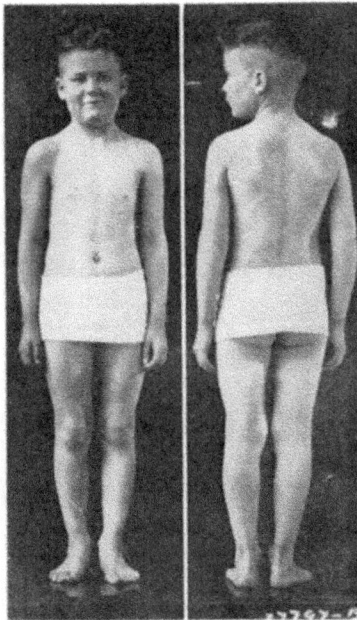

Fig. 2.   Evidence of optimal health in childhood.

Dr. Hugh Chaplin, chairman of the New York Nutrition Council, has compiled information which is extremely valuable in helping parents to judge whether their children are optimal (ideal) or just average, or possibly, defective.   A full discussion on this subject is given in the leaflet, "Signs of Health in Childhood."   (See references at the end of the booklet.)

The following are signs of health in childhood, compiled from this material.

A WELL BUILT BODY IS SHOWN BY:

1. *Hair*—Plentiful, with lustre due to sufficient natural oil.
2. *Eyes*—Bright and clear, no squinting, no dark fatigue rings under the eyes.   Membranes of the lids pink and free from inflammation.
3. *Unobstructed nasal breathing*—Ability to breathe deeply and easily thru the nose with mouth closed, especially when exercising or sleeping.
4. *Teeth*—Clean, strong, well enameled teeth, free from cavities, set in jaws wide enough to contain them without crowding. The grinding surfaces of the double teeth meet directly. The upper front teeth slightly overlap.

5. *Mucous Membranes*—Color of membranes of the mouth and eyes and also the color of the finger nails is definitely pink. (Richness of iron in blood.)

6. *Skin* — Slightly m o i s t, clear, and smooth.

7. *Muscles*—Firm and strong, with sufficient fat.

8. *Shoulders*—E v e n, f l a t shoulder blades. Not rounded forward. Head is held erect, chin in.

9. *Chest*—Broad and d e e p with good expansion (2-3 inches).

10. *Straight back and flat abdomen.*

11. *Arms and Legs* — L o n g bones are straight, not bowed out or inclined inward so that knees knock together. T h e joints are not enlarged.

12. *Ankles*—Inner and outer sides equally prominent. The tendon in the back of the heel should be straight.

13. *Feet*—Well arched a n d strong. Inner border is straight from heel to tip of big toe. Feet are parallel in standing or walking.

14. *Weight*—Proper w e i g h t for height, age and type a n d frame. Regular gain, small or heavy, at a satisfactory rate.

A BODY IN GOOD RUNNING ORDER IS SHOWN BY:

1. *Expression*—Happy a n d alert, cheerful disposition. (The close relationship between bodily and mental health cannot be too strongly emphasized.)

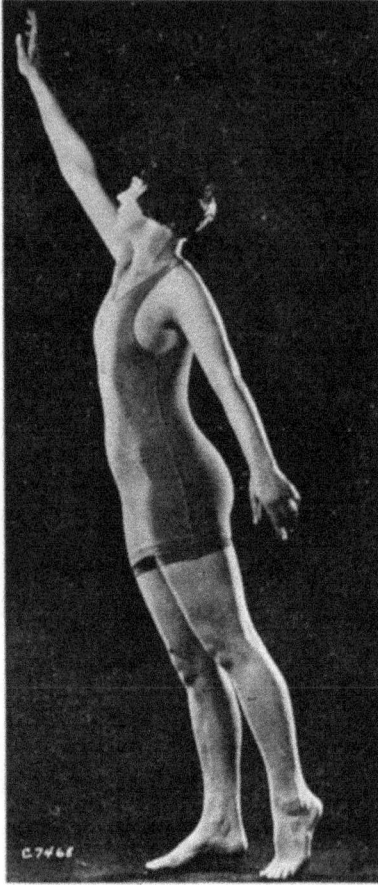

Fig. 3. Evidence of optimal health in youth.

2. *Tongue*—Moist, red and clean.

3. *Breath*—Sweet.

4. *Good Posture*—(See picture "Posture Standards, U. S. Children's Bureau.")

5. *Muscle Control*—Muscles should work together like a trained team. Some awkwardness during the first two or three years may be expected. At 11 to 14 years, due to the more rapid growth of arms and legs than of the trunk, there is a tendency to awkwardness which normally disappears a little later.

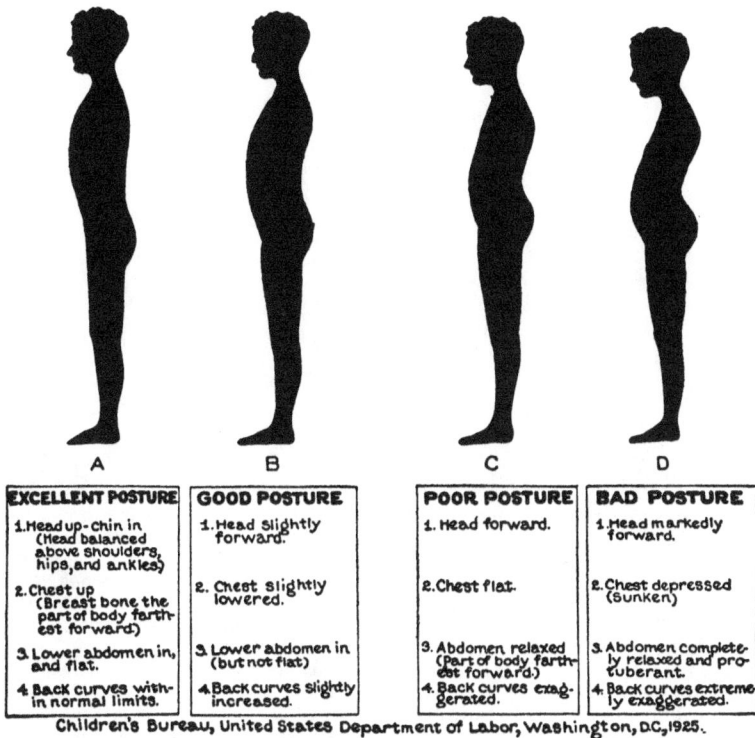

A	B	C	D
EXCELLENT POSTURE	**GOOD POSTURE**	**POOR POSTURE**	**BAD POSTURE**
1. Head up-chin in (Head balanced above shoulders, hips, and ankles)	1. Head slightly forward.	1. Head forward.	1. Head markedly forward.
2. Chest up (Breast bone the part of body farthest forward)	2. Chest slightly lowered.	2. Chest flat.	2. Chest depressed (Sunken)
3. Lower abdomen in, and flat.	3. Lower abdomen in (but not flat)	3. Abdomen relaxed (Part of body farthest forward.)	3. Abdomen completely relaxed and protuberant.
4. Back curves within normal limits.	4. Back curves slightly increased.	4. Back curves exaggerated.	4. Back curves extremely exaggerated.

Children's Bureau, United States Department of Labor, Washington, D.C., 1925.

Fig. 4. Differences in posture are due to differences in bone and muscle development and general vigor.

6. *Bodily Repose*—No nervous twitching or unnatural activity.
7. *Endurance*—No distress or undue fatigue on ordinary exercise.

III.   What We May Hope to Gain by Proper Food Habits

NORMAL GROWTH AND PHYSICAL DEVELOPMENT ARE DEPENDENT ON PROPER FOOD

It was thought in the past that differences in growth and development of children were largely due to climate, heredity and other factors and that nothing that we could do would alter growth. Dr. Emmett Holt has found that the children of Japanese and of Russian Jews who are born and raised in this country are both taller and heavier than those reared in Russia or Japan; he attributes this condition to the greater abundance of growth foods in the diets of the foreign children who are reared in America. Dr. Holt has observed, too, that the children of Americans of the most intelligent classes tend to run heavier and several inches taller than their parents; this condition he also attributes to the results of bettered practices in feeding and hygiene. While climatic conditions are still admitted to have an influence, such are no longer considered an all-important factor in

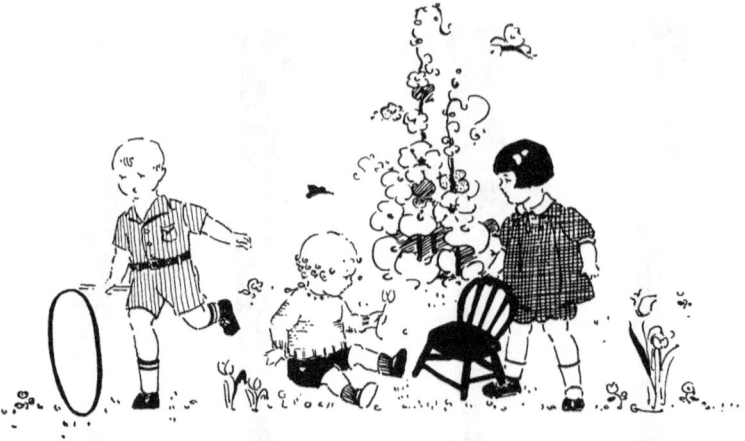

Fig. 5. Children, like flowers, need sunshine.

growth, altho it is conceded that some children inherit greater impetus to grow than others do. Dr. William R. P. Emerson offers the following from his wide experience with undernourished children:

"Time and again when a certain child has seemed pre-destined to be thin, because of an unmistakable resemblance to a thin forbear, we have seen him attain normal weight and maintain it with proper food and care." Also Dr. Emerson adds, "The thin grandfather is no longer accepted as sufficient reason for failure in nutrition."

Experiments with young animals have repeatedly shown that changing growth can be accelerated or retarded at will by changing the diet —all other conditions remaining the same. At present, this fact is so well established that it is standard practice in scientific research to determine the value of a diet by noting the extent of gain or loss in the animal's weight. For example, in testing the potency of cod liver oil for the growth, or the A vitamin, white rats of standard age, breeding, weight and environmental conditions are selected. Cod liver oil is fed in measured quantities with a diet in which vitamin A is supplied only by the oil. Under these conditions the rate of gain in weight shows the potency of a particular lot of the cod liver oil for its growth vitamin.

STRONG, STRAIGHT BONES AND PERFECT TEETH AND FREEDOM FROM RICKETS ARE THE RESULTS OF RIGHT FOOD AND HEALTH HABITS

1. *Rickets is a common disease of childhood.*
The well built body has been described previously. Unfortunately, the average person has several too many imperfections of bone and tooth structure which were preventable, had the mother understood how to safeguard the child in the prenatal period and the early years. However, this fact has been known for a few years only.

This disease of childhood, causing such commonly observed defects as knock knee, inturned ankles, a crooked back or breast bone, or crooked and protruding teeth, is called **rickets**.

2. *Definition of rickets.*
Rickets is defined as a disease in which there is failure to deposit the mineral elements which give hardness to the bones. Usually there

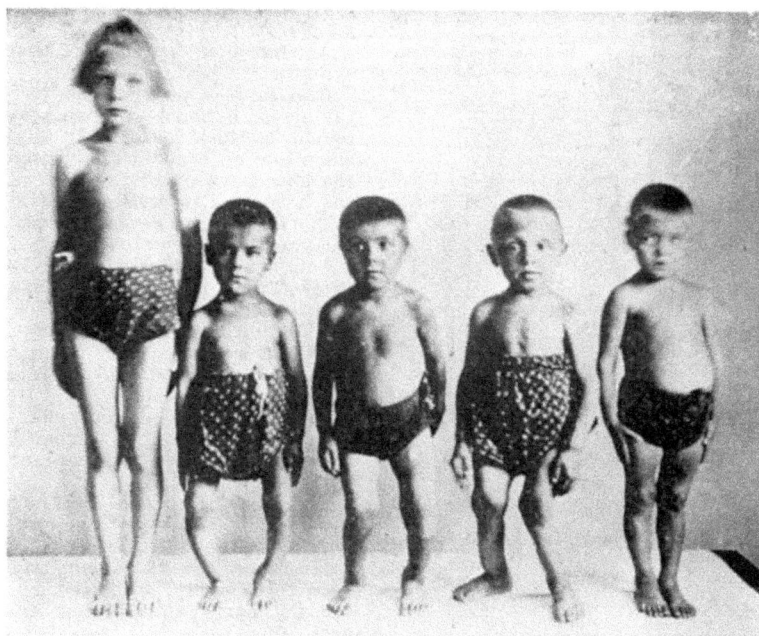

Fig. 6. Symptoms of rickets. All are seven-year-old children. The four on the right are stunted and deformed by rickets.

is found an over growth of cartilage at the ends of the long bones, causing large bulging joints. Also, the bones being soft, become bent and distorted. Some of the most common symptoms of rickets are easily seen by the parent if informed on the subject. In case several of the symptoms occur at the same time, the parent will suspect that all is not well and take measures to overcome the trouble. It is always wise to consult a reliable physician.

While rickets is not commonly considered fatal in itself, it weakens the body and pre-disposes to other diseases and this is a factor in infant mortality. As explained before, deformities may persist into adult life.

3. *Extent and occurrence.*

It is said by reliable authorities that from 50 to 75 percent of all children show mild to serious symptoms of rickets in infancy. The disease is most apt to occur in premature and in bottle-fed babies, tho breast-fed babies may be afflicted if the mother's hygiene and diet are poor during the prenatal and the nursing period. Twins are more apt to suffer than a single baby. It is most apt to occur in infants of from 7 to 12 months, and up to two years of age, altho a form known as "late rickets" may develop under extreme conditions at a more advanced age, as in the period of rapid growth in adolescence. More cases occur in winter than in summer. March and April are the months in which it appears most often, due to faulty diet and to winter housing and lack of direct sunshine. All groups of society are affected.

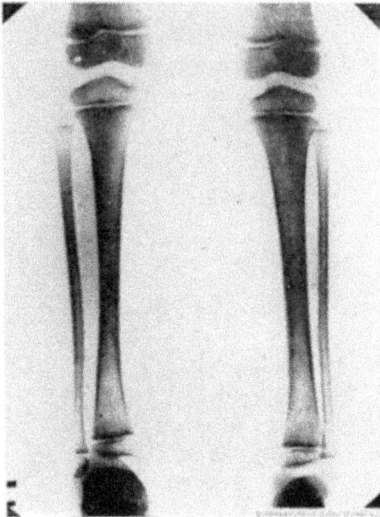

Fig. 7. X-ray picture of bones showing normal development.

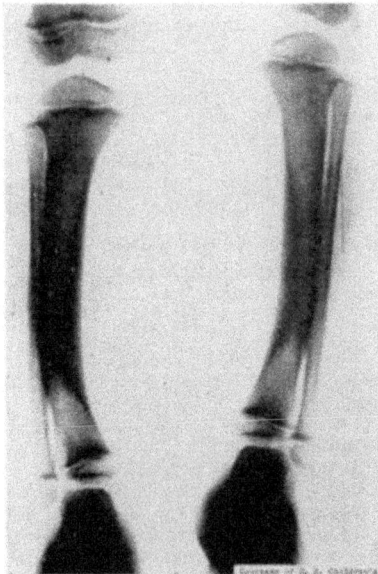

Fig. 8. X-ray picture of bones showing enlargements at the end and bending due to rickets.

4. *Symptoms of rickets (Compiled from various sources.)*

A. Nervous; usually the first symptom.

Restlessness, peevishness, fretful sleep, hypersensitiveness to touch, marked increase in perspiration, or head sweating and the hair worn off of the back of the head, due to restlessness.

B. Muscular; flabbiness and weakness.

Commonly evidenced in the protruding abdomen — "young robins' belly." The heart muscle has diminished power to accommodate to exercise; easy fatigue.

C. Bone defects due to failure to deposit calcium.

(1) Head. The fontanelles do not close properly. Normally these should close at about 18 months.

The frontal bones may be thickened, causing abnormal bulging of the forehead.

Misshapen head, causing the head to be square or flattened.

Jaws narrowed, forcing the arch upward. This interferes with the permanent teeth coming in straight and lessens nasal space, thus favoring adenoids. sometimes this deformity of the jaw may be so marked as to alter the features in an unbecoming way.

(2) Chest. Deformed, flattened. Ribs flaring. or with knob-like formations, "beading" sometimes called "rachitic rosary."

Crooked and protruding breast bone; called "pigeon breast."

Depression of the chest at the end of the sternum; called "funnel breast."

Shoulder blades protrude; "angel wings."

These conditions cause the lungs to become crowded, hindering them in development. This leads to lowered vitality and predisposes to respiratory diseases. Chest deformities are quite apt to persist into adult life.

(3) Trunk. Curvature of the spine. This condition may be exaggerated by poor posture as the

child grows older. The pelvic bones may become misshapen. It is generally agreed by scientists that difficulties in child-birth may arise in adult life from this cause.

(4) Limbs. Enlargements of the joints or fingers, wrists, knees and ankles may result. Frequently these enlargements at the wrists of infants are mistaken for fat by the parents. Bow legs and knock knees are common manifestations. The heavy child is more apt to show bow legs than a light one, because of added weight on soft bone. (In severe rickets, these deformities may persist into adult life.)

D. The mineral content of the bones and blood is shown by laboratory tests to be much diminished.

5. *Causes of rickets.*

Rickets has been developed in experimental animals in three distinct ways. Observation on children having the same disease shows that similar causes exist in the human family.

A. Lack of minerals in the diet. If the food of infants is lacking in the lime and phosphorus salts, or, if these elements are not in the correct ratio, the bones and teeth do not develop normally, due to the lack of proper building material. Patent baby foods, when these contain large amounts of sugar or starch, cause rickets because of the deficiency in mineral elements which the breast milk or properly modified cow's milk supplies. The older child's need of these minerals is taken care of with a quart of milk daily.

B. Lack of the vitamin D or rickets preventing element in the diet.

In this case something seems to be lacking which is necessary to proper utilization of minerals in bone and tooth structure. The difficulties in digestion may affect the child's ability to make use of calcium; foods best supplied with this element are cod liver oil, eggs and fresh leafy vegetables. Because cod liver oil is the best of all known

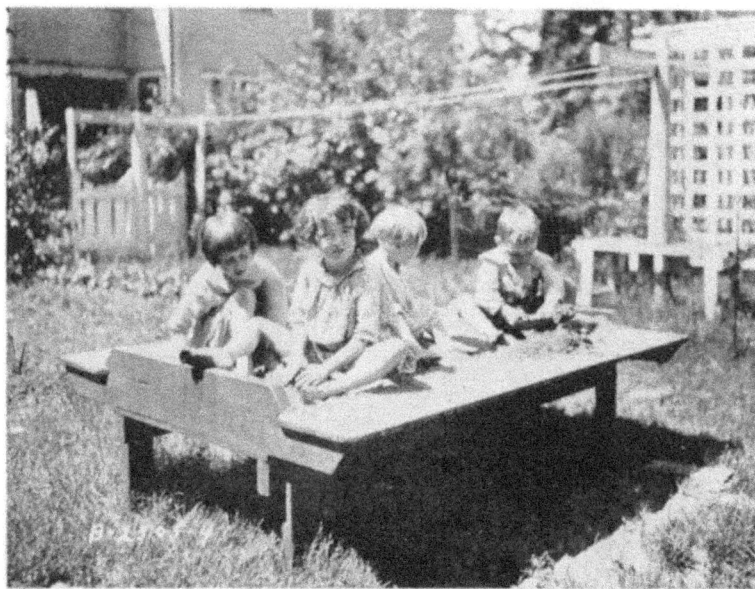

Fig. 9. Sunshine and outdoor play—an easy prescription for children to take.

foods for the rickets preventing element, it is considered a safety measure to include it in the baby's diet for the first year during the second and third winters, and at any other time when there is a tendency to colds, or growth is slow. Fall and winter babies, and bottle babies need special protection, beginning with five drops at one month and gradually increasing to 2 or 3 teaspoons daily at nine months of age (Dr. A. F. Hess). Usually the latter amount is sufficient for the older child or the adult who wishes protection from cold and to safeguard teeth.

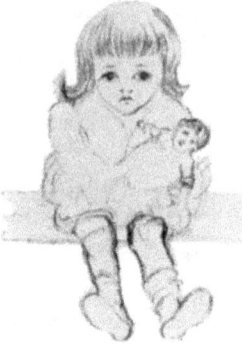

Eggs are especially good for the vitamin D element when the hen is having direct sunshine and green foods. This is one reason for includings eggs in the daily diet. Green leafy vegetables have been found to be valuable for the same purpose.

C. Lack of direct sunshine.

Exposure of the direct rays of the sun has been found to be an effective way to held the child to get lime in the bones and teeth and keep it there. The ultra-violet rays are known to be the potent rays.

Fig. 10. Malnourished child.*

These active rays of sunshine cannot pass thru ordinary window glass, clothes and air heavily laden with dust, but can pass thru quartz glass with practically no loss. Vita Glass, Cello-Glass and Flex-O-Glass are some of the substitutes which allow these active rays to pass in considerable amount and thus are good substitutes for ordinary window glass for windows in a sleeping or play room, or on a sun porch.

All children (and adults) should get as much direct sunshine as possible without actual sunburn. An even coat of tan on the body without burn is much to be desired. Said one mother newly enlightened on the value of sunshine, "I used to try to keep my children from getting tanned. Now I see how brown their bodies can become during the summer."

All children may benefit by a minimum of clothing and a maximum of outdoor play in the summer sunshine. Bathing suits or sun suits that are sleeveless and short legged, bare feet or shoes and short socks, are not only comfortable but healthful.

6. *Age periods needing special protection against rickets.*

Experiments have shown that the mother who has proper food and direct sunshine during

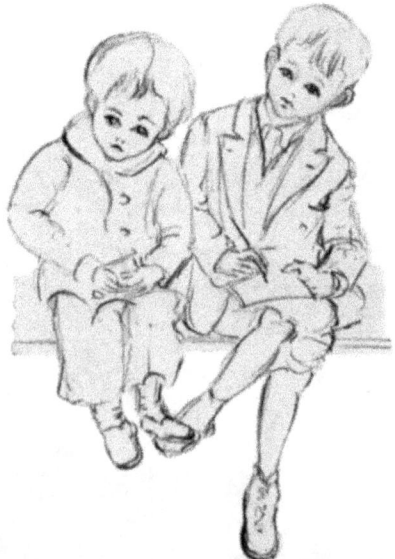

Fig. 11. Evidence of malnourishment.*

*Observe serious expression of these children, quite unlike the expression of happy, well children of normal weight. Sketches by Joanne M. Hansen, Head of Applied Art, Iowa State College. Children of Brittany, France.

pregnancy and nursing will help to protect her baby from the development of rickets and promote good tooth structure in her child.

Children up to 6 years and again at about 10 to 16 years grow most rapidly and. therefore. are apt to exhaust their calcium supply. Adolescent rickets may develop during the later period of 10 to 16 years.

7. *Diet and sunshine safeguard teeth.*

Since rickets and tooth defects are found to be due to the same causes, the principles which apply in preventing and curing rickets, also safeguard the teeth in their development and are an important factor in preserving them. This applies to adults as well as to growing children.

Some interesting observations have been made in New Zealand upon the frequency of dental decay among school children, due to diet. It was shown that the nearer the candy stores were to the schools, the greater the number of decayed teeth found in the pupils. Also it was discovered that children who were given pocket-money, which was largely spent for sweets, had poorer teeth than children whose parents were too poor or who did not allow this indulgence.

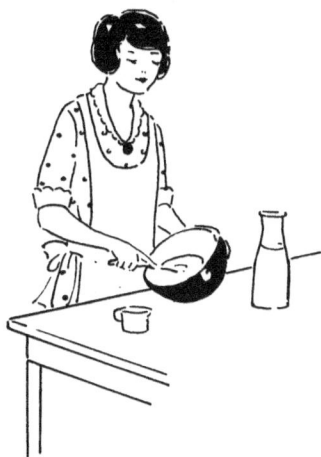

Fig. 12. Problems of appetite and digestion are best solved in the kitchen.

To provide all the dietary essentials for sound teeth, the average diet should include:

(a) More milk and milk products and more eggs.
(b) More whole grain products and less white flour.
(c) More fruits and tomatoes and less sugar.
(d) A goodly quantity of leafy vegetables.
(e) More raw and uncooked foods.
(f) Coarser foods that cleanse the teeth.
(g) Hard foods to exercise the jaws in chewing.

Exposure of the body to the sun's rays or small doses of cod liver oil will enable the body to make full use of the lime in the diet. (For further information on this topic, refer to special mimeograph leaflet, "Bone and Tooth Defects in Children," A-1262).

A GOOD APPETITE AND DIGESTION AS WELL AS FREEDOM FROM CONSTIPATION WILL BE ASSURED WITH PROPER FOOD

Lack of appetite, upsets in digestion, and constipation are commonly reported by mothers as childhood problems with which they must contend. If the suggestions for feeding the child which are given in the pamphlet, "Essentials in the Daily Diet," are consistently followed, these problems should not occur. In case the constipation habit has been formed, the condition can be overcome in almost all instances with proper diet without the aid of laxatives or physics.

The following suggestions should prove helpful in overcoming constipation:

1. Foods with special laxative properties. Most fruits—especially figs and prunes. Vegetables—especially the fresh or green leafy ones and onions and carrots. Cereals, oatmeal, cracked wheat, prepared

bran, shredded wheat, graham or rye bread. Natural sugars as honey, molasses, maple sugar. Ordinary buttermilk, or culture buttermilk, as acidolphilous milk have special laxative qualities.

2. Foods for bulk or roughage:
Fruits, vegetables and bran of cereals. Agar-agar may be used in addition to these foods.

3. Plenty of water:
One or more glasses before breakfast and between meals. Lemonade.

4. General habits to form:
Good mastication.
Movement of bowels twice daily at a regular time.
Plenty of sleep and rest.
Vigorous play out of doors.
Freedom from worry and excitement.
Special exercises to correct constipation.
No physics. Mineral oil, or petrol-agar for temporary use only.
(For further help on constipation see special mimeograph leaflet, Constipation, CT-2).

THERE IS BETTER PROGRESS IN SCHOOL WHEN THE CHILD IS PROPERLY NOURISHED AND GROWING NORMALLY.

Recent studies of school children show that there is a close relationship between rapid physical growth (evidence of good nutrition) and school progress. Dr. Bird T. Baldwin, State University of Iowa, has collected data on school children in this country and abroad which shows that generally:

1. Dull pupils are shorter and lighter than bright or average pupils.

2. The tall, heavy boys and girls with good lung capacity are more mature physically as well as more mature mentally (as shown by school progress) than are short, light-weight boys and girls.

A study of 80,662 children in the Detroit public schools showed that children below grade for age were generally shorter and lighter than the average child of that age. Children above grade or age were generally taller and heavier than the average child of that age. These facts indicate that there is a close relationship between physical and mental conditions and that the mind has increased power to function when nutrition is good.

Dr. Smiley Blanton at present of Vassar College, made observations on 6500 school children in Germany during the recent war. About 40 percent of these children were found to be suffering from malnutrition. Mental and nervous symptoms were reported as follows:

Lack of energy, easily fatigued mentally and physically.

Inattention, difficulty in concentration.

Poor memory.

Slow comprehension, longer to think.

Unusual restlessness, could not sit still.

Unusually dull and quiet, seemingly mentally stupid.

These facts show why the malnourished child makes poor progress in school and that the effect of the body on the mind is quite as marked as the effect of the mind on the body.

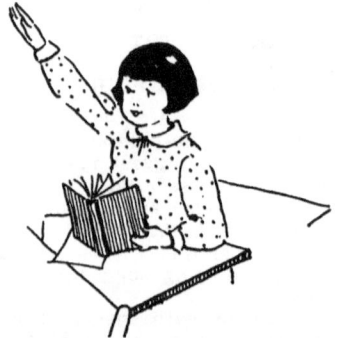

Fig. 13. The well-nourished child makes better progress in school.

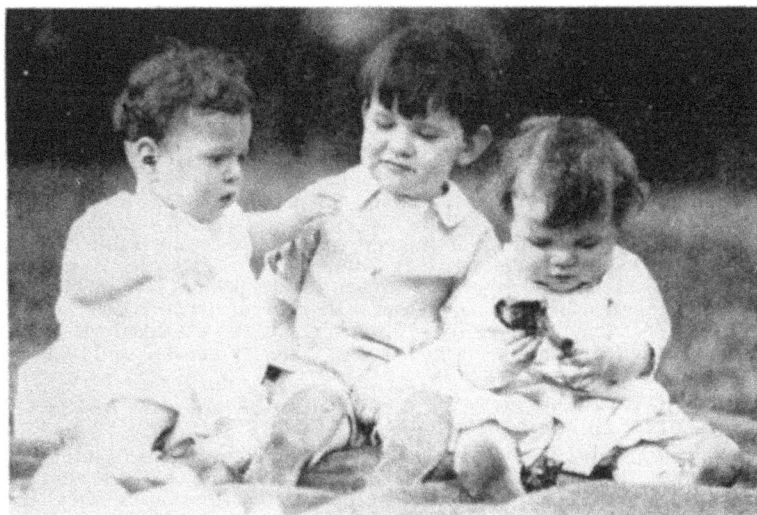

Fig. 14. Well-fed children offer better resistance to disease.

THE PROPERLY FED CHILD IS HAPPIER AND BETTER BEHAVED.

Many of us have observed the well fed baby to be one that is happy and interested in what goes on about him, while the poorly nourished infant is apt to be fretful, irritable and nervous. With the older child as with the infant which is suffering from malnutrition, there is a shrinking away from normal interest and activity and the "no" attitude develops. This negative attitude is the result of fatigue or illness due to poor nutrition as well as faulty habit training. If malnutrition persists, the ultimate effect will be a child with a bad disposition. A feeling of well-being is the foundation on which to build a good disposition and a cheerful outlook on life.

THE WELL NOURISHED CHILD OFFERS BETTER RESISTANCE TO DISEASE.

In experiments with laboratory animals, which are fed on poor diets, there is a very high mortality from infectious diseases. For example, many of the animals which are given a diet deficient in the A vitamin, die from "colds" and respiratory or glandular infections before developing the eye disease, which is characteristic of this food deficiency. In contrast, animals on good diets are remarkably free from infections of various kinds.

Similar effects to the above mentioned were noted on children during the recent war. When many children in Europe suffered from an extreme lack of the proper kind or amount of food, there was a very high mortality from infectious diseases, but only a very few cases of actual starvation. The poorly nourished child is an easy victim of disease and is, therefore, often characterized as "catching everything that comes along." (This may include the too fat as well as the too thin child.) Many times an undernourished child will take one infection after another and sometimes succumb to their combined effects, while a robust child under the same conditions will be unaffected. Susceptibility as well as exposure to disease, determines whether the child will have the catching disease. Building up resistance thru proper food will safeguard the child from many infectious diseases and other ills.

FREEDOM FROM ANEMIA.

Following infections such as influenza, pneumonia, measles, or in case of loss of considerable blood, or with prolonged faulty food and hygiene, and from many other causes, there is a tendency to anemia (lack of red corpuscles and iron in the blood). Proper food is not only a preventative but a cure for most cases of anemia. Even pernicious anemia, which was thought formerly to be incurable, within recent years has been found to respond to diet; especially if a large quantity of liver, which seems to act as a specific for anemia, is included in an otherwise good diet. In general, such a diet is one well balanced and high in liver, iron, and all the essential vitamins (For further information on such a diet, refer to special Child Training mimeograph on Anemia.)

CONTROL OF OR RECOVERY FROM DISEASE MAY BE LARGELY OR WHOLLY DEPENDENT ON RIGHT FOODS.

Diabetes is one of the diseases which is considered due to improper eating. In this disease the hope for a comfortable existence or of prolonged life is largely dependent on strict attention to diet, tho heredity is said to enter into the problem.

In cases of prolonged fever, such as typhoid, the rapidity or the chances for recovery will depend largely on sufficient highly nourishing foods being supplied in an easily assimilated form. The same may be said of such conditions as ulcers of the stomach or of other highly irritated or abnormal conditions of the digestive tract. (For further information refer to Child Training mimeographs on "Food Values That Diabetics Should Know" and "Non-Irritating Diets.")

THE CHILD THAT IS PROPERLY FED POSSESSES A MORE VIGOROUS AND MORE BEAUTIFUL BODY.

This point is so well understood that it needs no emphasis, for strength and beauty are the results of right habits of living. The well built body and the body in good running order, which have been described previously, is a strong and beautiful body. The parent who knowingly permits the sacrifice of the child's health, strength and perfection of body to weak indulgence of the child in vicious foods, is handicapping him for future success and happiness in life. Surely no parent would wish to be guilty of such serious neglect.

Let us keep in mind the well-developed, optimal child as the ideal for which we are striving: Well-developed bones, good posture and chest development; strong, even, white teeth; firm muscles, and sufficient well-distributed fat; skin that is clear and free from blemish, showing the ruddy glow of health; hair smooth and glossy; dry clear eyes with no dark circles underneath; mouth kept closed, breathing only thru the nose; the mind alert and active; the disposition good, full of high spirits, and not irritable or restless.

The rewards of right eating are mental and physical fitness. For food we spend the largest part of our income in money and time. The market basket may be your best ally and not your enemy in attaining the desired goal of physical perfection and abounding health and vigor in your child.

> There is one lesson at all times and places,
> One changeless truth on all things changing writ
> For boys and girls, men, women, nations, races—
> Be fit—be fit! And once again, be fit!
> —Rudyard Kipling.

The Child's Bill of Rights

The ideal to which we should strive is that there shall be no child in America that has not been born under proper conditions, that does not live in hygienic surroundings, that ever suffers from under-nutrition, that does not have prompt and efficient medical attention and inspection, that does not receive primary instruction in the elements of hygiene and good health; that there shall be no child that has not the complete birthright of a sound mind in a sound body and the encouragement to express in fullest measure the spirit within which is the final endowment of every human being.—Herbert Hoover, Chairman, American Child Health Association, New York.

Questions

1. What is the general difference in the "average" and the "optimal" well child?
2. State 10 evidences of a well-built body.
3. State 5 evidences of a body that is in good running order.
4. To what extent is heredity responsible for growth and physical development?
5. What is rickets? Name conditions favoring the disease.
6. What are the symptoms of rickets?
7. State three causes of rickets?
8. Name two foods that are used to prevent rickets. By what methods can you provide more sunshine?
9. How does food affect appetite? Elimination? Disposition?
10. How is food important in building up resistance to colds? Control of anemia? Diabetes?

References

BOOKS:

*Holt, Dr. Emmett, M. D.: "Food Growth and Health".
Nutrition in its relation to progress in school, and to resistance to disease.

McCollum, E. V., Ph. D.: "The Newer Knowledge of Nutrition."
3rd Edition. Diet in relation to teeth. Chap. I. p. 472-493.
The Nutrition of the Suckling. Chap. 22, p. 451. Diet and
Resistance to Disease, p. 531.

*Emerson, Wm. R. P., M. D.: "The Child, His Nature and His
Needs."
The Relation of Nutrition to Mental Development. Chap. 9,
p. 159.

Mendel, Lafayette, B., Ph. D.: "Nutrition, the Chemistry of Life."
Vitamins. Chap. 3.

*Lucas, William Palmer: "The Health of the Run-about Child."

Peters, Lulu Hunt: "Diet for Children."
The Malnourished Child. p. 157-171.
Goiter, Rickets, Tuberculosis, Skin Disorders. p. 207-222.

*Books in traveling library.

Emerson, Wm. R.: The Intellectual Giant Is Not a Physical
Dwarf.
Delineator, Feb., 1926.

PAMPHLETS:

"Food, Teeth and Health." The Child Federation of Philadelphia.

"Nutrition Picture Stories." Iowa State College.

"Children's Teeth." Iowa State University at Iowa City.

Kenyon, Josephine H., M. D.: "A Special Letter on Sterility,"
Good Housekeeping Magazine, 119 W. 40th, New York City—
15 cents.

Chapin, Hugh, M. D.: "Signs of Health in Childhood."
American Child Health Ass'n, 370 7th Ave., New York City—
25 cents.

"Sun Babies," Children's Bureau, Washington, D. C. leaflet. Free.

Iowa State College Extension Service:
"Bone and Tooth Defects in Children," Mimeograph A-1262.
"Constipation," Mimeograph CT-2.
"Anemia," CT-42.
"Food Values that Diabetics Should Know," CT-16.
"Non-Irritating Diets," CT-23.

Cooperative Extension Work in Agriculture and Home Economics, Iowa State College of Agriculture and Mechanic Arts and the United States Department of Agriculture cooperating. Extension Service, R. K. Bliss, Director, Ames, Iowa. Distributed
in furtherance of the Acts of Congress of May 8 and June 30, 1914.

Child Care & Training Booklets

Toys and Play

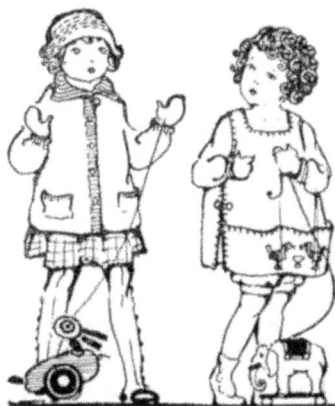

IOWA STATE COLLEGE
EXTENSION SERVICE

Toys and Play

By Mrs. Alma H. Jones

Christmas, in the minds of children, is synonymous with toys, for at this season it has long been the custom of parents and others to make gifts of toys to their children. Since most children are more interested in play than anything else, a toy naturally suggests itself, when, at the Christmas Season, the occasion arises for a gift which will bring joy and happiness to little ones.

Wise and Unwise Gifts of Toys

Too often these gifts, so well intended, are selected unwisely, since the average adult thinks of toys only as a source of pleasure and pastime. Beyond a consideration of the price he wishes to pay and the pleasure he wishes to give, the benevolently inclined adult usually sees little else to be considered in making a purchase. Sometimes the parent is influenced solely by the child's desires and begging. A child who is surrounded in the toy shop by a riot of color, noises and many ingenious mechanical devices is likely to desire those that have the greatest immediate appeal and not to choose those that will eventually give the most lasting pleasure when once he uses them. The wise parent will distinguish between the child's passing whim and his vital interest in toys just as he resists the temptation to allow too much sweets or too many movies.

Not long ago, a group of nursery school children aged one and a half to three years were seen selecting their own toys for a period of play. Free choice was given them of such playthings as toy animals in great variety, dolls, beads, blocks, etc., with which they were used to playing each day. Six of the 10 children chose the blocks with which they played the entire period. Because they had experienced the satisfactions given by blocks in a variety of shapes and sizes in previous play periods, they chose these promptly from among the other things which seemingly offered more appeal. Had these children lacked previous experience with blocks, or if they had been surrounded by clever displays of ingenious devices of all kinds, arranged to attract the prospective buyer of toys, they probably would not have been able to make a wise choice under these conditions.

While it is true that many temptations are offered today to buy cheap and harmful novelties in toys, the opportunity to select really fine and useful toys has never been better, if we know how to make use of it.

Toys should give pleasure and bring joy and happiness but, at the same time, they should assist in the education of the child in body, mind and character. Since character building is the aim and end of education, toys should be considered as material which serves this purpose, and we should seek to discover what qualities in toys best further this end.

Tests for Desirable Toys

"Toys, real toys, are the tools of play." Here are some of the standards by which we can judge the desirability of toys.

1. TOYS MUST BE SAFE

Particularly, in buying toys for the small child, it is imperative that safety be given first consideration. There must be no tacks, such as are often used for eyes in teddy bears, or small bells and buttons which can be pulled off and swallowed by the infant. Practically all toys for the baby should be washable, since he invariably puts everything in his mouth. All painted or dyed articles must be non-poisonous and fast in color. Lacquer finish which permeates the wood will not chip off as frequently does enamel paint.

Hair on dolls and dogs which becomes dirty with use may be a source of danger. Guns may be dangerous and foster carelessness in the use of firearms. Generally, for this reason they should be avoided altogether as playthings. Military toys that create the spirit of destructiveness and foster callousness in the value of human life should be discouraged. For small children avoid toys that make startling noises and sudden movements.

2. TOYS MUST BE DURABLE IN MATERIAL AND WORKMANSHIP

Any toy that soon pulls to pieces is a poor purchase from the standpoint of expenditure of money; no matter how small the original cost. Since such toys are too flimsy for proper care and repair they encourage extravagance and destructiveness, while really worth while toys which resist wear and which are kept in repair encourage thrift and conservation of property.

3. TOYS SHOULD BE ARTISTIC IN FORM, COLOR AND EXPRESSION

The child's appreciation of color, form, sounds and his attitude toward things and people will be greatly affected by his earliest toys. For this reason, toys should be simple in design, harmonious in color and genuine in expression. Avoid poorly proportioned and ugly shapes, simpering expressions (as on dolls), inharmonious colors and harsh, jangling noises. Harsh, metallic sounds from toys are not only unpleasant for the family to live with but unwholesome in their effect on the child. Rattles and toy musical instruments should be chosen for their pleasing sounds. When buying a toy musical instrument, such as a zylaphone, (a very commendable toy) one should observe whether it produces the scale in a fairly true manner, otherwise leave it in the toy shop if you value your child's development in musical appreciation.

4. TOYS SHOULD BE ADAPTED TO THE AGE AND THE CONTINUED USE OF THE CHILD

When the baby first begins to stare at objects and grasp them, he is old enough for toys. The good toy should adapt itself to new uses in more complicated ways as the child grows older. Blocks are one of the best examples of play material which adapts itself to the successive stages of development of the child. As a tiny infant, he will enjoy grasping and staring at bright colored blocks. Later, he gets much pleasure from handling them, putting them in a basket and dumping them out again. At about two years he will enjoy fitting blocks into a special box made for that purpose and making towers or trains of several together. From three to six years he begins to enjoy arranging the various colored blocks to make simple designs, while blocks of assorted sizes and shapes will be used to build imaginative trains, towers, bridges, etc. Dolls, clay crayons and blackboard, colored beads and tinker toys are other examples of toys which are adapted to different uses as the child grows older.

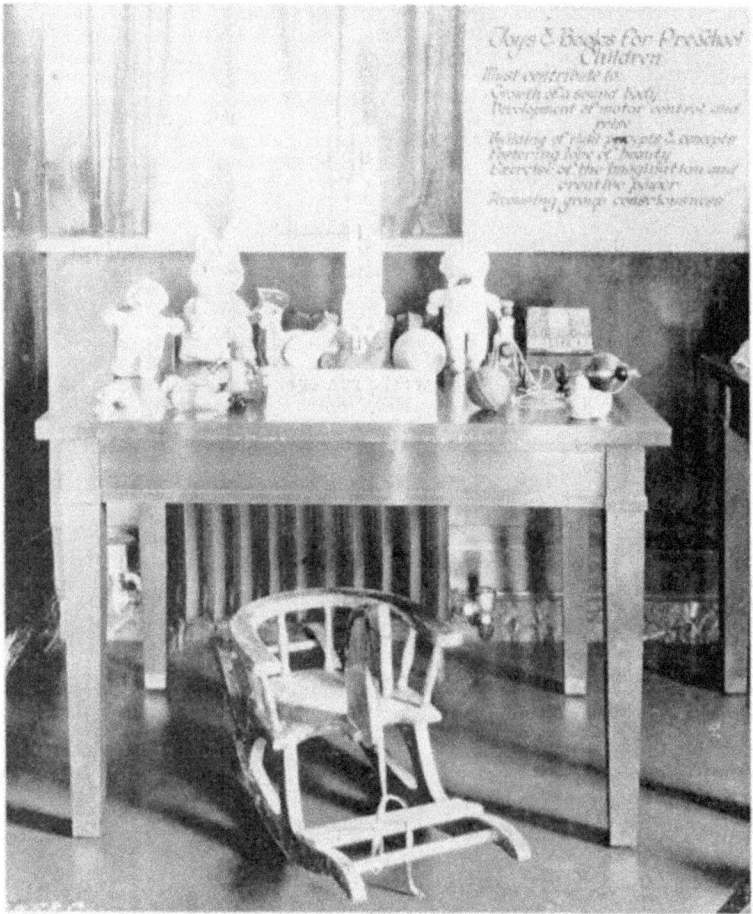

Fig. 1. Toys for the littlest ones.

Toys for Different Ages

1. TOYS FOR THE BABY

Toys for the baby should help to train his senses and to develop his large muscles. Many articles commonly found in every home give the baby his greatest pleasure; spools, clothes pins, large wooden spoons, pie tins and potato mashers are favorites.

Some toys which may be bought and which are acceptable are simple rattles, (small, brightly colored gourds are good) rubber dolls, floating bath toys, soft 'cuddly' dolls and teddy bears. Large brightly colored rubber balls that roll from him and require his efforts to recover them again are a safe means of encouraging the child to walk.

2. FOR THE TODDLER

When the child begins to walk, at an average age of about 13½ months, he needs toys that encourage active play both indoors and outdoors. Push and pull toys now are especially good. The "follow-me" tinkers that don't turn upside down are a boon to the busy mother.

Sand tables and sand piles with pails, bottles, scoops and measures of various kinds are a source of lasting pleasure and benefit, for thru their use he is learning muscle control and is getting ideas regarding weight, measure, form, texture, etc. Kiddie cars, express wagons, wheelbarrows and garden implements give him healthful outdoor play and develop muscle-control.

Indestructable picture books, balls, colored beads, large crayolas, tinker toys and large peg boards provide wholesome indoor play which furthers the development of his senses and of his muscles.

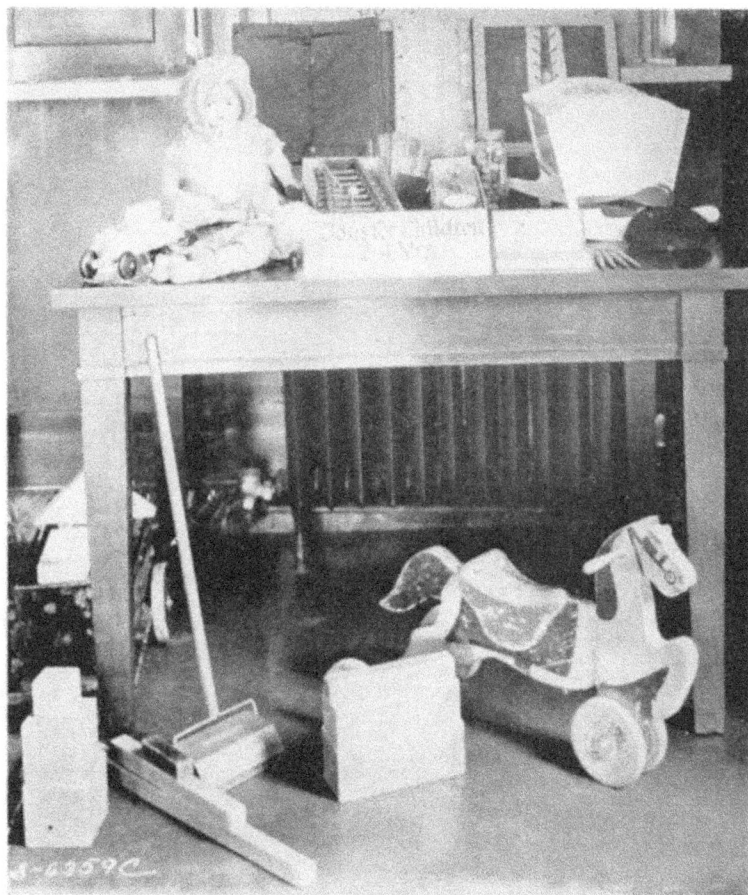

Fig. 2. Toys for children, 2 to 4 years.

3. FROM THREE TO SIX YEARS

Toys and play for this period should continue to develop the larger muscles and, to a certain extent, the more delicate ones. Since the imagination is developing rapidly at this time, children should have many *free materials—"do with" toys with which things can be constructed.* In general, boys and girls interests should not be differentiated at this early age. We need not be afraid of making boys "sissy" by allowing them to play with dolls, or of making "tomboys" out of our girls by giving them an express wagon.

Besides the things mentioned for the previous age, the following are desirable: Tricycles, swings, ropes to climb on and to jump, footballs, hammer, nails and saw (small size with good cutting edge). Be sure, however, that supervision is given the use of the saw in the beginning, unless you wish to risk having such things as the piano bench ruined or the neighbor's sapling tree cut down.

Large sized blocks and such equipment as dolls, dishes, furniture, laundry equipment, water colors (non-poisonous) and brushes, blunt scissors and colored paper, blackboards and chalk, and clay for modelling are excellent for indoor play.

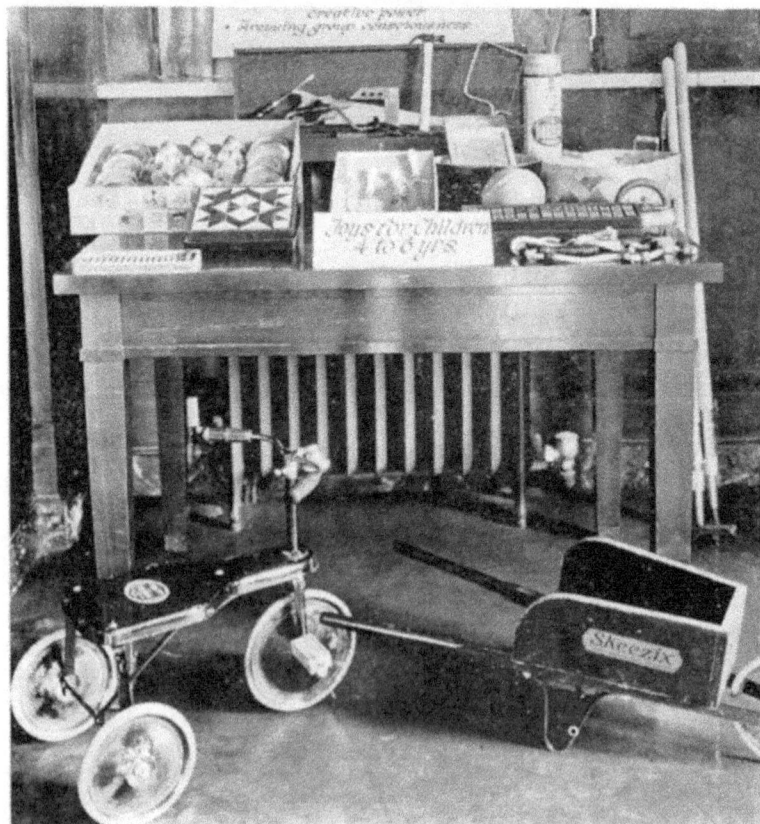

Fig. 3. Toys for children, 2 to 6 years.

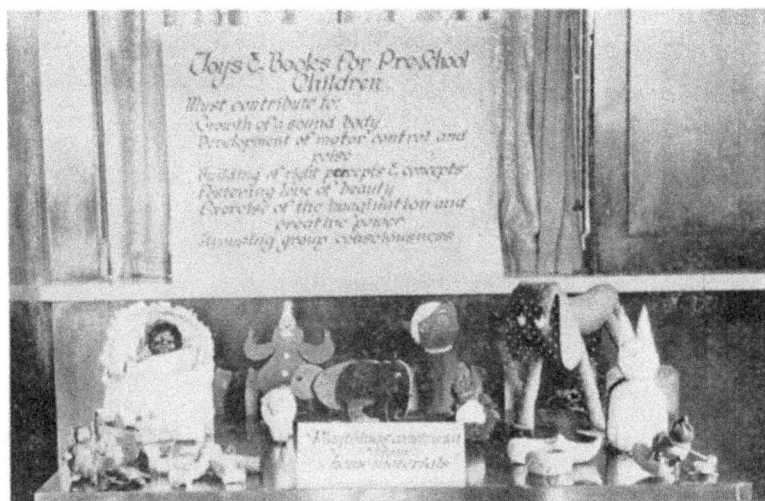

Fig. 4. Playthings made of home materials.

In general, mechanical devices in which the toy does all the work and the child does nothing offer no chance for creative work and foster idleness and a desire to be amused on the part of the child. The normal child will soon tire of such a toy and take it to pieces to see how it works. To quote Kate Douglass Wiggins, "Everyone knows that the simple natural playthings which are nothing more than pegs on which a child hangs his glowing fancies are healthier than our modern mechanisms in which the child has only to press the button and the toy does the rest."

4. THE SCHOOL CHILD

Children from 6 to 12 years should have toys that satisfy their love of activity and their desire for sports and games. Girls will continue to find much interest in dolls and housekeeping equipment, but they should be encouraged also in sharing outdoor or athletic interests with boys. In buying sports equipment buy only things of good quality and suited to the purpose it is to serve, such as the following: Footballs, baseballs and bats, tennis balls and rackets, roller and ice skates, (shoes attached) fishing tackle and scout knives. Sports clothing such as sweaters, hiking boots, boy scout and camp fire girl outfits are a good addition to the sports equipment listed. Further additions may be made to the carpentry equipment as special saws, work-bench, vise, etc., depending on the youngsters interest. Games of all sorts, as they develop self-dependence in thinking and action, train the child in cooperation in group activities are commended. Equipment which encourages interest in scientific experimentation such as chemistry or radio outfits are splendid.

Apparatus for home and back yard:

HOME:

Small table, chairs with low straight backs.
Low shelves for toys.
Horizontal bars in doorway.
Sand table.

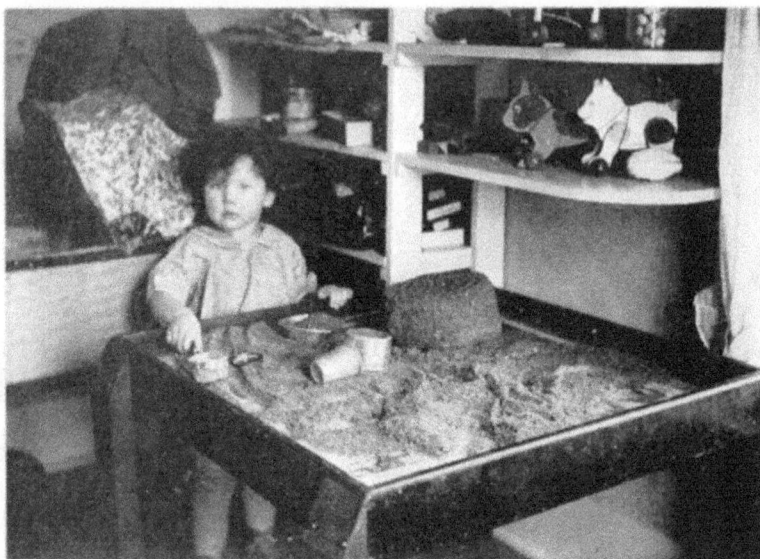

Fig. 5. A homemade sand table provides many hours of wholesome play.

YARD:

Sand pile and a space to dig, or a garden.
Swings, made of rope or discarded casings.
Slide.
Walking boards, ladders.
Climbing rope.
Empty boxes, blocks, bricks.

Making the Most of Toys and Play in Character Training

Good habits or bad habits may be fostered in the use of toys. Some of the desirable traits which may be fostered thru the wise use of toys and play activities are:

1. Neatness and orderliness thru care in the use of playthings, as sweeping spilled sand or water, and in putting toys away.
2. Thrift in the wise purchase and repair of playthings.
3. The habit of keeping wholesomely busy. (The idle child is the one who gets into trouble by constantly looking for amusement provided by others.) The mechanical toy may develop love of being entertained.
4. Purposive thinking and activity in construction and dramatization with play objects often carries over into creativeness in adult life.
5. Concentration and control of the will thru attempting one thing at a time and accomplishing it. "Sticking at the job" is easy when the child is interested, as in his play.
6. Interests may be awakened which will carry over into achievement in adult life. For example, the early experimental play of Thomas Edison formed the basis of later scientific discoveries.
7. Cooperation and ability to get on with others may be fostered thru sharing in sports and games, and "playing the game" according to the rules.

8. Good manners may be taught effectively thru play. For example, the tea set and the tea party may provide the setting and occasion for teaching table manners, as the dolls must be versed in accepted table manners and social customs.

9. Love and sympathy for others may be fostered thru imitation of the sympathetic attitude toward dolls.

10. The sense of ownership may be taught thru having playthings and a play space which are respected by other children and adults. Respect for "mine" and "thine" is fostered in the child thru having certain possessions of his own and likewise being bound to respect others' possessions.

11. The right opportunity is provided for showing off, as the child can show what he can do, not how he looks.

12. Ability to think and reason correctly is fostered thru gaining first hand knowledge in active play.

13. Knowledge and skill may be acquired with toy equipment that will be useful in adult work, e. g., housekeeping, cookery, carpentry, etc.

Making Things from Home Materials

Many common or waste materials found in every home, and nature materials, which abound around country homes, have the greatest possibilities for "making things." Children should be encouraged to use such materials for play and experimentation.

Too much emphasis should not be placed on the finished product, as the expression of the child's own ideas (creativeness) is of greater importance than the utility of the play thing, altho gradual improvement in workmanship may be expected without too much adult supervision.

Especially, on rainy days, children will enjoy the use of such materials as follows: (Fill in other uses than those mentioned where possible.) (Meek, 6).

1. WASTE MATERIAL.
   Newspapers or wrapping paper.
   Cutting soldier caps, pinwheels, costumes, paper dolls.
   Paper Bags.
   To blow up for balloons, masks, kites, Japanese lanterns, postman bags.
   Mailing tubes.
   Horns, jumping rope handles, dolls.
   Paper boxes.
   Wagons, furniture, houses, lanterns, street cars, circus wagons, mail boxes, with oatmeal boxes for drums, silos, pull toys.
   Various kinds of paper.
   Wallpaper for May baskets, baskets, book covers, cut out patterns, paper for doll house.
   Corrugated paper for house roof, washboard.
   Tissue and lace paper for valentines, doll dresses.

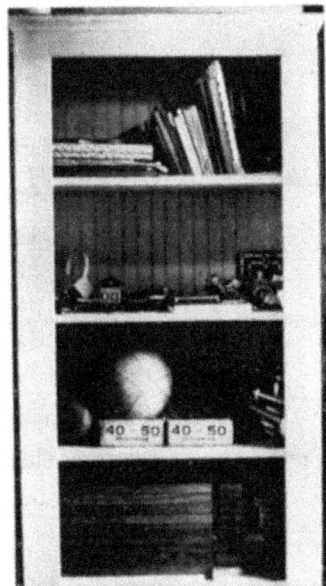

Fig. 6. A handy cupboard for children's playthings.

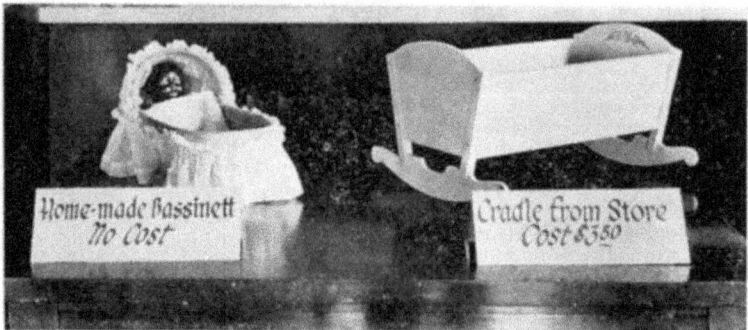

Fig. 7. Playthings often may be made of waste materials in the home.

Tinfoil, for Christmas tree decorations.
Parrafin paper, for drinking cups.
Paper towels, for paper dolls, art paper.
Magazines.
Material for scrap books, room decoration.
Bottles.
Bottle dolls, vases which are painted or covered with paper.
Scraps of cloth, felt.
For doll clothes and doll house furnishings.
Oil cloth, for scrap book covers, dolls, animals, etc.
Terry cloth towelling, for stuffed dolls, animals, etc.
Rope, cord, twine, rags.
Reins, jumping ropes, rugs, hammocks.
Corks.
For bath toys.
Spools.
Dolls, furniture, wheels.
Clothes pins.
Fences, dolls.
Button molds for wheels.

2. NATURE MATERIAL AND ITS USES:
Dandelions and clovers, for chains.
Seeds, for beads.
Milk weed pods, for cradles or boats.
Burrs, for animals, dolls, houses.
Pine cones for necklaces, Christmas tree decorations.
Corncobs, for dolls, fences.
Shells, for boats, necklaces.
Acorns, for dishes, tops.
Leaves of trees, for making hats.

3. CLAY:
Poking, pounding and rolling.
Modelling.
Marbles, dishes, beads, candle sticks, reproduction of objects.

4. WOOD:
Scraps of soft wood, for hammering nails, sawing, building of boats, carts, houses, etc. Odds and ends of different sizes and shapes for home made blocks.
(Plane and sandpaper, if necessary, to avoid splinters.)
Empty boxes, as grocery and chalk.
Cigar boxes for sand pile dolls.

5. BEAVER BOARD FOR TOY ANIMALS.
   The coping or jig saw may be used to cut these.
6. BRICKS AND STONES.
   All types of construction work.
7. PAINT.
8. RUBBER TUBES for woven mats, dolls, etc.

Economy in Toys and Play Material

1. Use all the home material possible.
2. Avoid too many toys, which encourage extravagance.
3. Buy durable toys that will last for a family of children.
4. Buy only a part of a set of blocks or tools or building material and add to them as the child grows older.

Questions

1. How are toys related to character education?
2. State four tests for desirable toys.
3. What purpose should toys serve in babyhood? The toddler? Pre-school age? Examples.
4. What is the advantages of "free material" versus "mechanical toys." Illustrate.
5. Name toys suitable to girls and boys of school age.
6. State five ways that good habits may be formed thru the proper use of toys and play.
7. Tell what uses children make of so-called waste material in play.
8. Suggest ways that you may use to provide a place for play and play materials.
9. Tell why construction or creative play with "free materials" is more than mere entertainment for children.

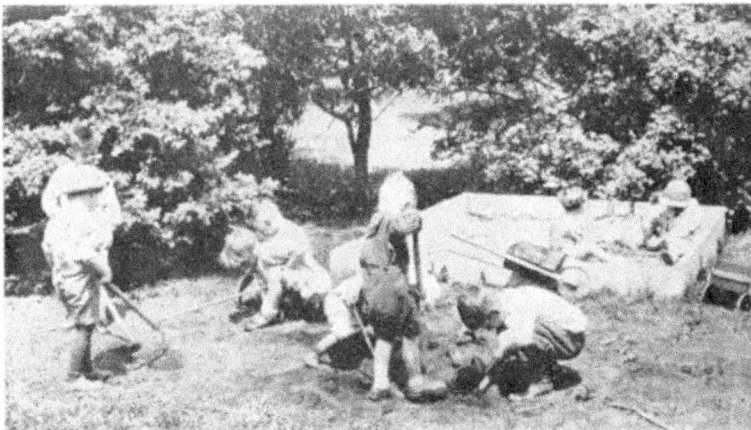

Fig. 8. Plenty of outdoor play is necessary to health.

References

1. Batchelor, W. C., "Home Play Bulletin No. 205."
   (Playground and Recreation Ass'n of America, 315 4th Ave., New York City, price 15c.)
2. Boyd, Neva L., "Play Equipment for the Nursery."
   (Chicago Ass'n. of Day Nurseries, 308 N. Michigan Ave., Chicago, price 10c.)
3. Garrison, Charlotte G., "Permanent Play Material for Young Children" (Scribner's 1926) Introduction.
4. Haviland. Mary S., "Character Training in Childhood", Chapter III, IV and V.
5. Leonard, Minetta S., "Best Toys for Children and Their Selection."
   (Wisconsin Kindergarten Ass'n, Madison, Wis., price 35c.)
6. Lucas, William P., "The Health of the Runabout Child," Chapter IX.
7. Meek, Lois H., "Interests of Young Children," price 10c.
   (American Ass'n. of University Women, 1634 Eye St., Washington, D. C.)
8. Norsworthy, N., & Whitley, Mary T., "Psychology of Childhood," Chapter XIII.
9. "Playthings," 20c.
   (Bureau of Ed. Experiments, 144 W. 13th St., New York.)
10. "Play and Recreation," Bulletin No. 92, 20c.
    (Government Printing Office, Washington, D. C.)
11. Backyard Playgrounds, Folder No. 2, 5c.
    (Children's Bureau, Washington, D. C.)

Catalogs giving current prices of play equipment may be obtained from these firms:

Wooden animals, blocks, etc.—A. Schoenhut Co., Philadelphia, Pennsylvania.

Color Cubes—Embossing Company, Albany, N. Y.

Kindergarten beads, pegs, pegboards, manila drawing paper, crayolas, large pennies, water colors—Thomas Charles Co., 2249 Calumet Ave., Chicago, Ill.

Playground Apparatus—Playground Equipment Company, 342 Madison Ave., New York.

Tables and Chairs—American Seating Company, Des Moines, Iowa.

Blocks—Pendleton & Townsend, Patterson, New York.

ACKNOWLEDGEMENT: Part of this material was originally printed in Wallace's Farmer, December 10, 1926 in the article "Timely Tips for Old Santa Claus," by the same author.

Cooperative Extension Work in Agriculture and Home Economics, Iowa State College of Agriculture and Mechanic Arts and the United States Department of Agriculture cooperating. Extension Service, R. K. Bliss, Director, Ames, Iowa. Distributed in furtherance of the Acts of Congress of May 8 and June 30, 1914.